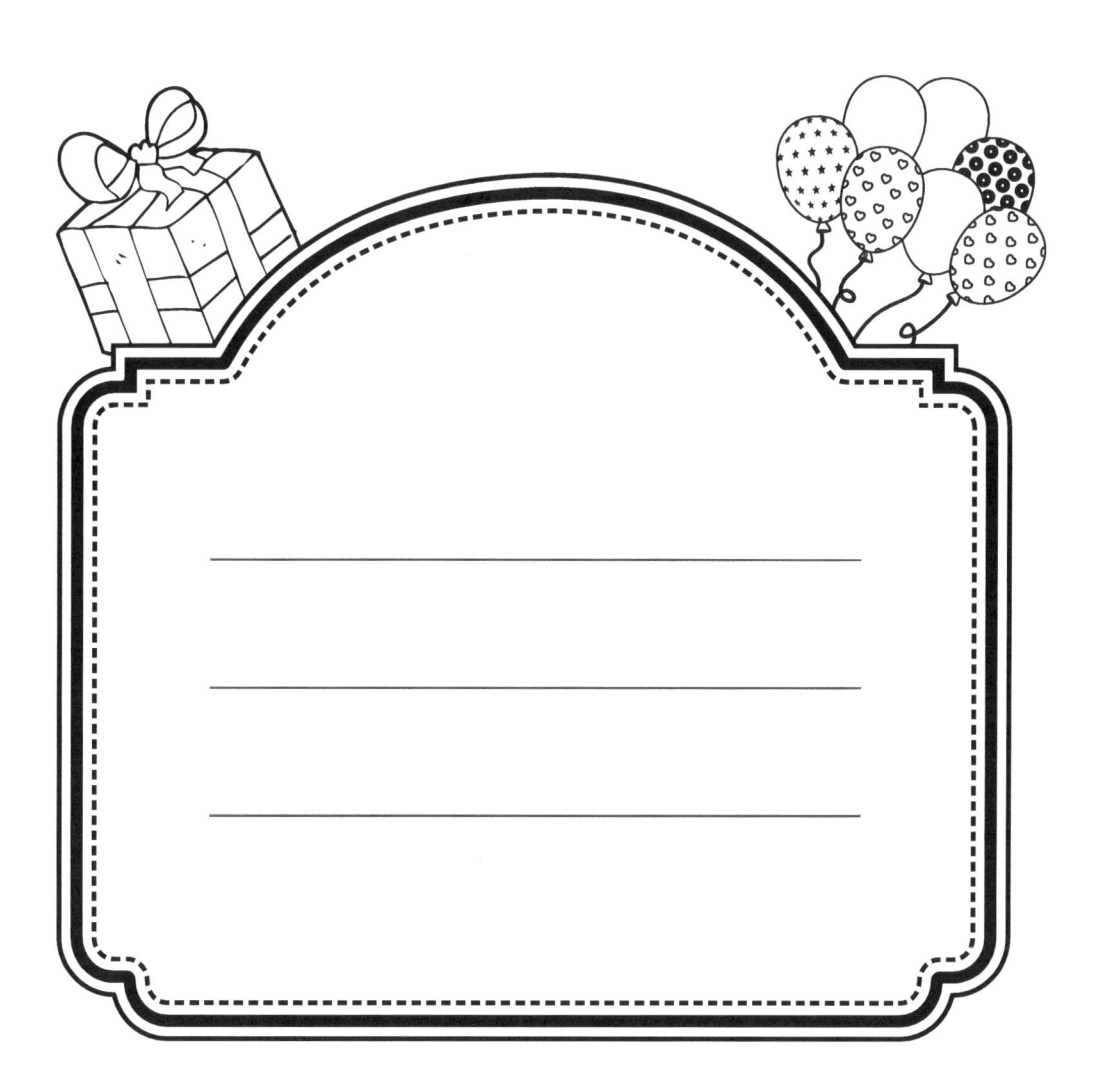

Guests

Name and relationship to parents

_____
_____

Advice for parents

_____
_____
_____

Wishes for baby

_____
_____
_____

Guests

Name and relationship to parents

_____

_____

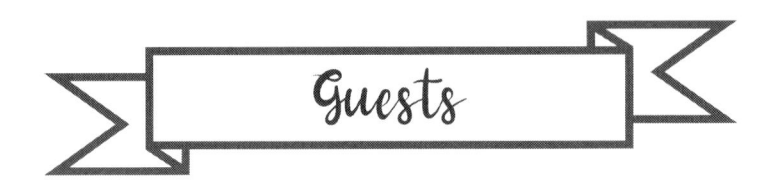

Advice for parents

_____

_____

_____

Wishes for baby

_____

_____

_____

Guests

Name and relationship to parents

_____
_____

Advice for parents

_____
_____
_____
_____

Wishes for baby

_____
_____
_____
_____

Guests

Name and relationship to parents

_____
_____

Advice for parents

_____
_____
_____

Wishes for baby

_____
_____
_____
_____

Guests

Name and relationship to parents

_____
_____

Advice for parents

_____
_____
_____
_____

Wishes for baby

_____
_____
_____
_____

Guests

Name and relationship to parents

_____
_____

Advice for parents

_____
_____
_____

Wishes for baby

_____
_____
_____
_____

Guests

Name and relationship to parents

_____
_____

Advice for parents

_____
_____
_____

Wishes for baby

_____
_____
_____
_____

Guests

Name and relationship to parents

_____

_____

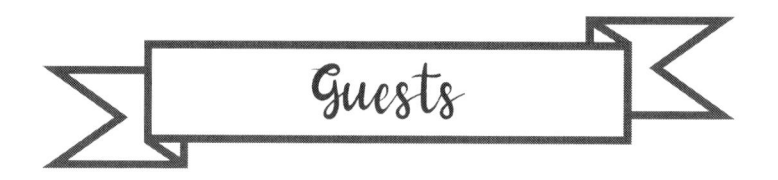

Advice for parents

_____

_____

_____

Wishes for baby

_____

_____

_____

Guests

Name and relationship to parents

_____
_____

Advice for parents

_____
_____
_____

Wishes for baby

_____
_____
_____

Guests

Name and relationship to parents

_____
_____

Advice for parents

_____
_____
_____
_____

Wishes for baby

_____
_____
_____
_____

Guests

Name and relationship to parents

_____
_____

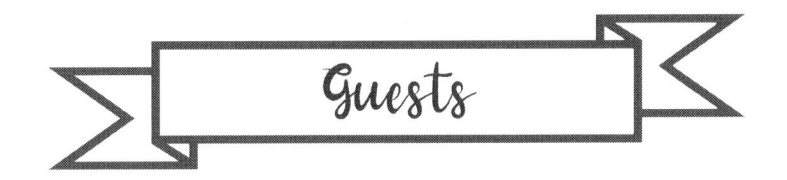

Advice for parents

_____
_____
_____

Wishes for baby

_____
_____
_____

Guests

Name and relationship to parents

_____

_____

Advice for parents

_____

_____

_____

_____

Wishes for baby

_____

_____

_____

_____

Guests

Name and relationship to parents

_____
_____

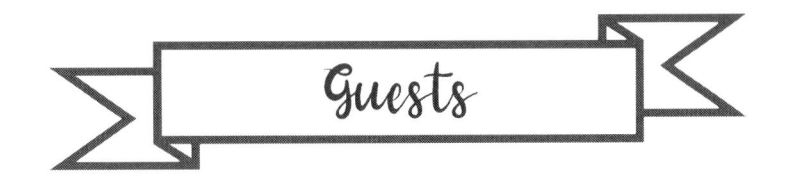

Advice for parents

_____
_____
_____

Wishes for baby

_____
_____
_____

Guests

Name and relationship to parents

_____

_____

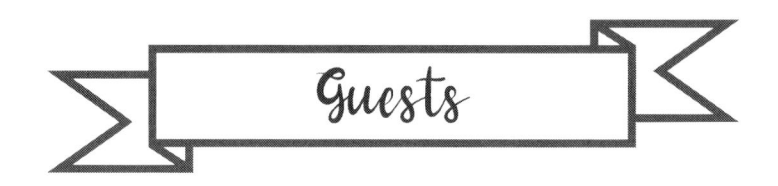

Advice for parents

_____

_____

_____

Wishes for baby

_____

_____

_____

_____

Guests

Name and relationship to parents

_____
_____

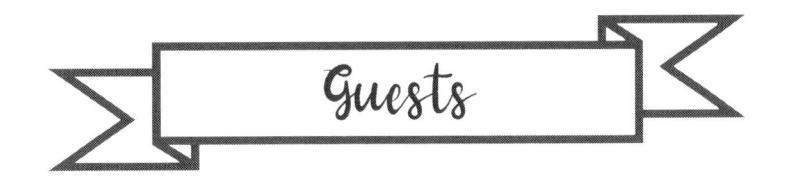

Advice for parents

_____
_____
_____

Wishes for baby

_____
_____
_____

Guests

Name and relationship to parents

_____

_____

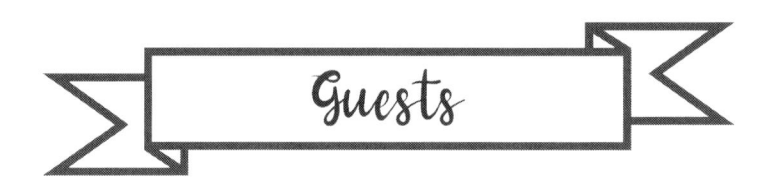

Advice for parents

_____

_____

_____

_____

Wishes for baby

_____

_____

_____

_____

Guests

Name and relationship to parents

_____
_____

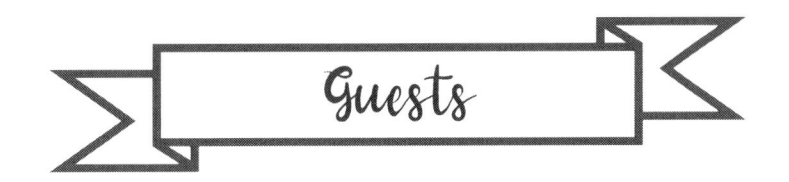

Advice for parents

_____
_____
_____
_____

Wishes for baby

_____
_____
_____
_____

Guests

Name and relationship to parents

_____
_____

Advice for parents

_____
_____
_____

Wishes for baby

_____
_____
_____

Guests

Name and relationship to parents

_____
_____

Advice for parents

_____
_____
_____
_____

Wishes for baby

_____
_____
_____
_____

Guests

Name and relationship to parents

_____

_____

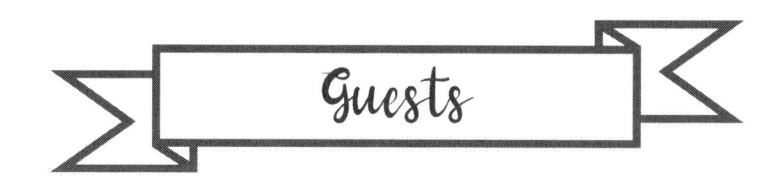

Advice for parents

_____

_____

_____

_____

Wishes for baby

_____

_____

_____

_____

Guests

Name and relationship to parents

_____
_____

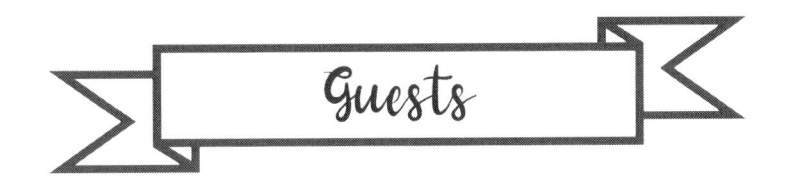

Advice for parents

_____
_____
_____
_____

Wishes for baby

_____
_____
_____
_____

Guests

Name and relationship to parents

_____
_____

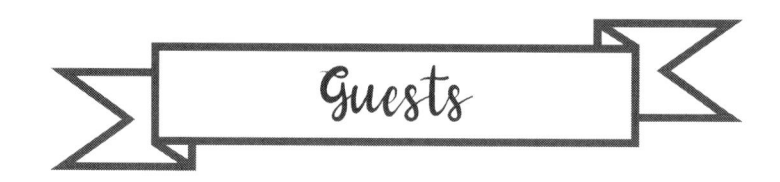

Advice for parents

_____
_____
_____

Wishes for baby

_____
_____
_____

Guests

Name and relationship to parents

_____
_____

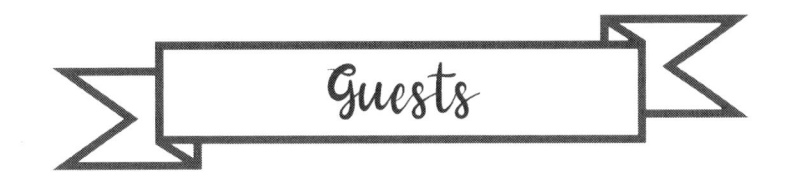

Advice for parents

_____
_____
_____

Wishes for baby

_____
_____
_____

Guests

Name and relationship to parents

_____
_____

Advice for parents

_____
_____
_____

Wishes for baby

_____
_____
_____

Guests

Name and relationship to parents

_____
_____

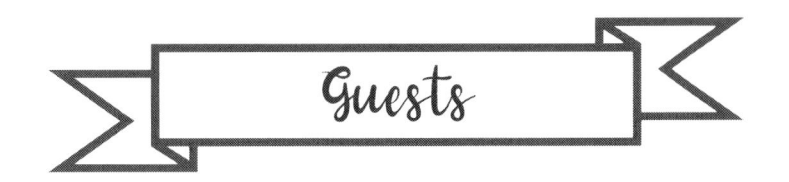

Advice for parents

_____
_____
_____
_____

Wishes for baby

_____
_____
_____
_____

Guests

Name and relationship to parents

_____
_____

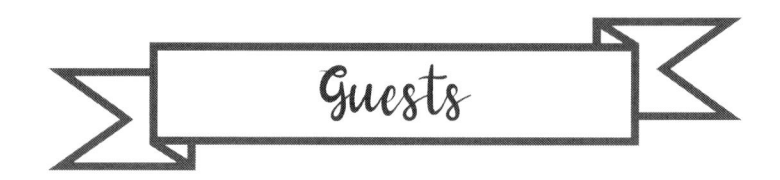

Advice for parents

_____
_____
_____

Wishes for baby

_____
_____
_____

Guests

Name and relationship to parents

_____
_____

Advice for parents

_____
_____
_____

Wishes for baby

_____
_____
_____

Guests

Name and relationship to parents

_____

_____

Advice for parents

_____

_____

_____

_____

Wishes for baby

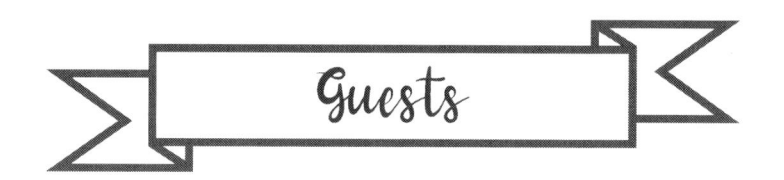

_____

_____

_____

_____

Guests

Name and relationship to parents

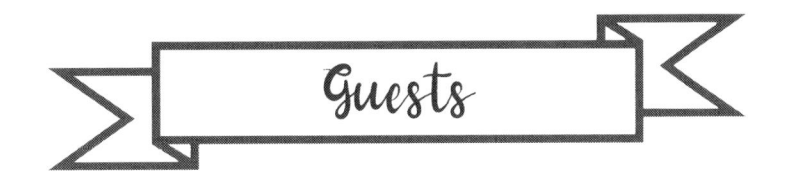

_____
_____

Advice for parents

_____
_____
_____

Wishes for baby

_____
_____
_____

Guests

Name and relationship to parents

_____
_____

Advice for parents

_____
_____
_____
_____

Wishes for baby

_____
_____
_____
_____

Guests

Name and relationship to parents

_____
_____

Advice for parents

_____
_____
_____

Wishes for baby

_____
_____
_____

Guests

Name and relationship to parents

_____

_____

Advice for parents

_____

_____

_____

_____

Wishes for baby

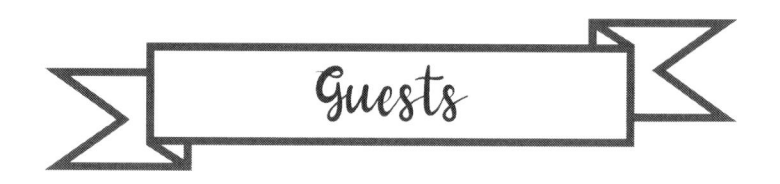

_____

_____

_____

_____

Guests

Name and relationship to parents

_____

_____

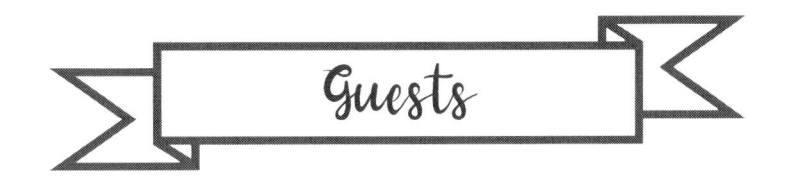

Advice for parents

_____

_____

_____

Wishes for baby

_____

_____

_____

Guests

Name and relationship to parents

_____
_____

Advice for parents

_____
_____
_____
_____

Wishes for baby

_____
_____
_____
_____

Guests

Name and relationship to parents

_____
_____

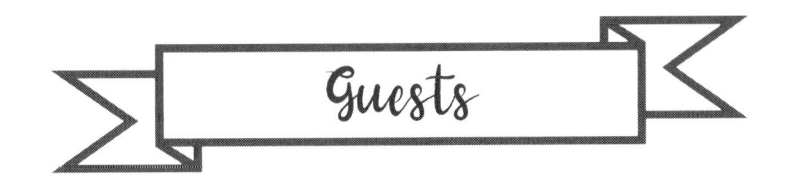

Advice for parents

_____
_____
_____

Wishes for baby

_____
_____
_____

Guests

Name and relationship to parents

_____

_____

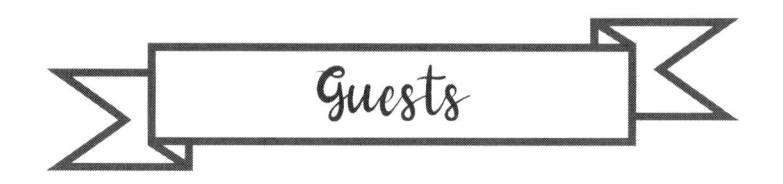

Advice for parents

_____

_____

_____

Wishes for baby

_____

_____

_____

Guests

Name and relationship to parents

_____
_____

Advice for parents

_____
_____
_____

Wishes for baby

_____
_____
_____

Guests

Name and relationship to parents

_____

_____

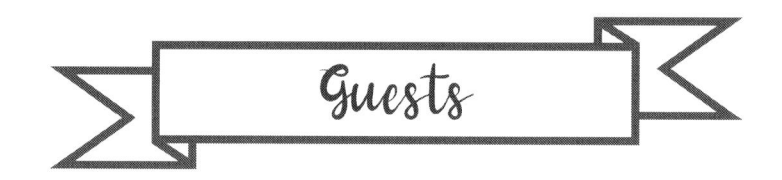

Advice for parents

_____

_____

_____

_____

Wishes for baby

_____

_____

_____

_____

Guests

Name and relationship to parents

_____
_____

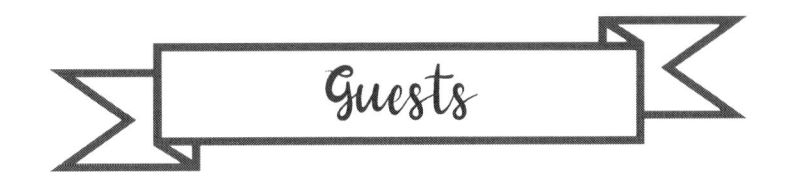

Advice for parents

_____
_____
_____
_____

Wishes for baby

_____
_____
_____
_____

Guests

Name and relationship to parents

_____
_____

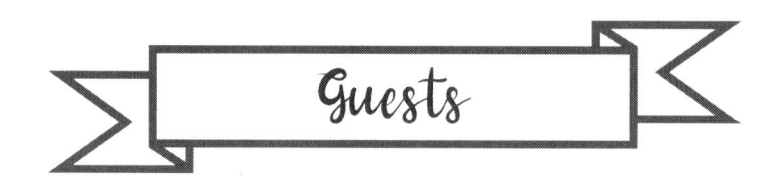

Advice for parents

_____
_____
_____

Wishes for baby

_____
_____
_____

Guests

Name and relationship to parents

_____
_____

Advice for parents

_____
_____
_____
_____

Wishes for baby

_____
_____
_____
_____

Guests

Name and relationship to parents

_____

_____

Advice for parents

_____

_____

_____

Wishes for baby

_____

_____

_____

Guests

Name and relationship to parents

_____
_____

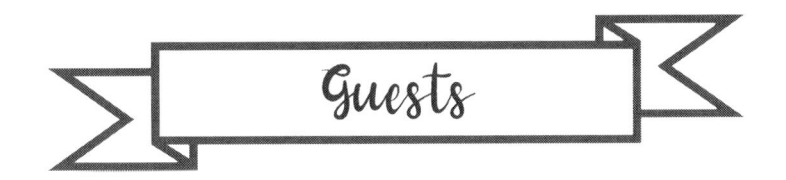

Advice for parents

_____
_____
_____

Wishes for baby

_____
_____
_____

Guests

Name and relationship to parents

_____
_____

Advice for parents

_____
_____
_____

Wishes for baby

_____
_____
_____
_____

Guests

Name and relationship to parents

_____
_____

Advice for parents

_____
_____
_____

Wishes for baby

_____
_____
_____
_____

Guests

Name and relationship to parents

_____
_____

Advice for parents

_____
_____
_____
_____

Wishes for baby

_____
_____
_____
_____

Guests

Name and relationship to parents

_____
_____

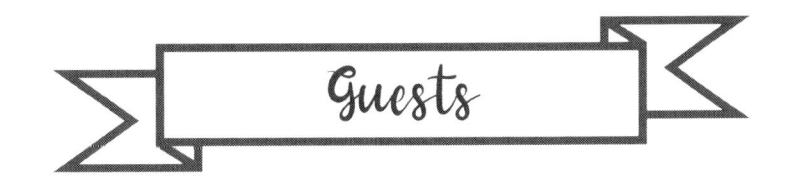

Advice for parents

_____
_____
_____

Wishes for baby

_____
_____
_____

Guests

Name and relationship to parents

_____
_____

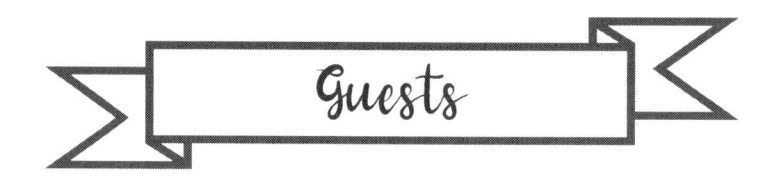

Advice for parents

_____
_____
_____

Wishes for baby

_____
_____
_____

Guests

Name and relationship to parents

_____
_____

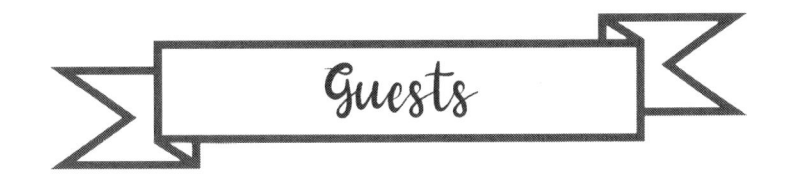

Advice for parents

_____
_____
_____

Wishes for baby

_____
_____
_____

Guests

Name and relationship to parents

_____
_____

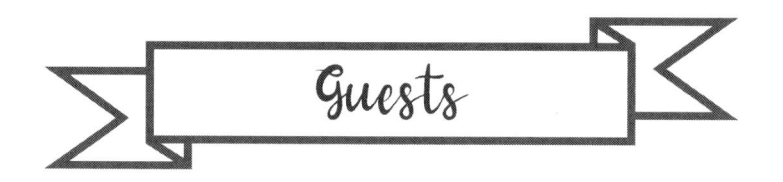

Advice for parents

_____
_____
_____
_____

Wishes for baby

_____
_____
_____
_____

Guests

Name and relationship to parents

_____
_____

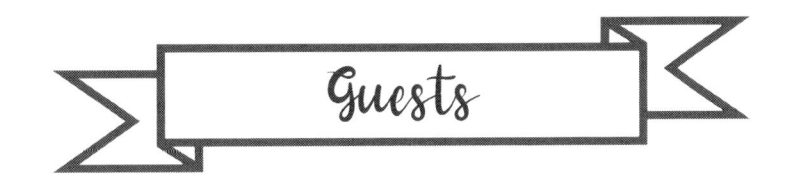

Advice for parents

_____
_____
_____

Wishes for baby

_____
_____
_____

Guests

Name and relationship to parents

_____
_____

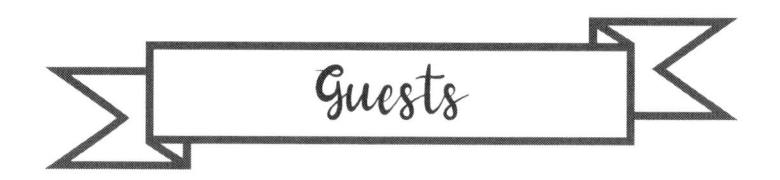

Advice for parents

_____
_____
_____
_____

Wishes for baby

_____
_____
_____
_____

Guests

Name and relationship to parents

_____
_____

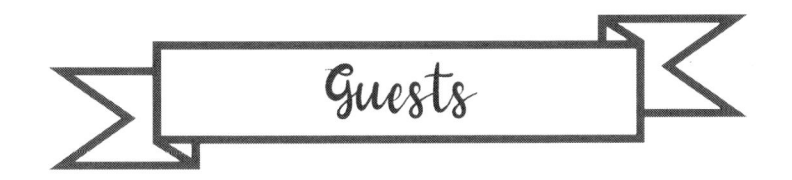

Advice for parents

_____
_____
_____

Wishes for baby

_____
_____
_____

Guests

Name and relationship to parents

_____

_____

Advice for parents

_____

_____

_____

Wishes for baby

_____

_____

_____

Guests

Name and relationship to parents

_____
_____

Advice for parents

_____
_____
_____

Wishes for baby

_____
_____
_____

Guests

Name and relationship to parents

_____
_____

Advice for parents

_____
_____
_____

Wishes for baby

_____
_____
_____

Guests

Name and relationship to parents

_____
_____

Advice for parents

_____
_____
_____
_____

Wishes for baby

_____
_____
_____
_____

Guests

Name and relationship to parents

_____

_____

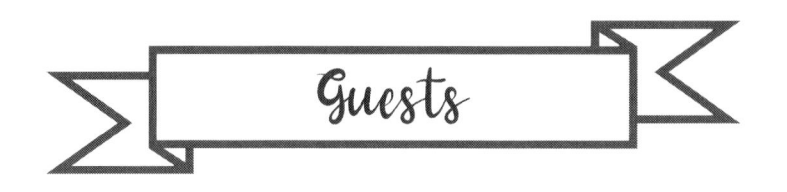

Advice for parents

_____

_____

_____

Wishes for baby

_____

_____

_____

Guests

Name and relationship to parents

_____
_____

Advice for parents

_____
_____
_____

Wishes for baby

_____
_____
_____

Guests

Name and relationship to parents

_____
_____

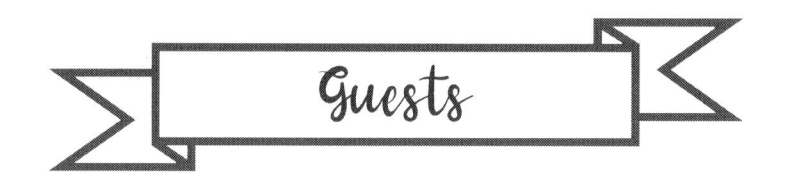

Advice for parents

_____
_____
_____
_____

Wishes for baby

_____
_____
_____
_____

Guests

Name and relationship to parents

_____

_____

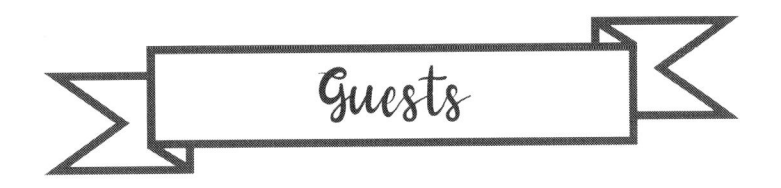

Advice for parents

_____

_____

_____

Wishes for baby

_____

_____

_____

Guests

Name and relationship to parents

_____

_____

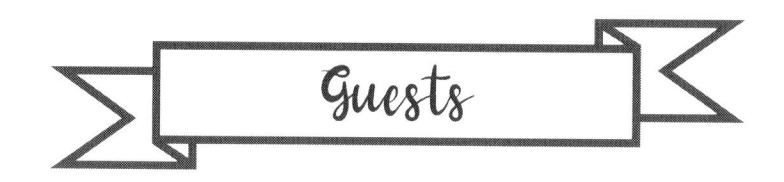

Advice for parents

_____

_____

_____

_____

Wishes for baby

_____

_____

_____

_____

Guests

Name and relationship to parents

_____
_____

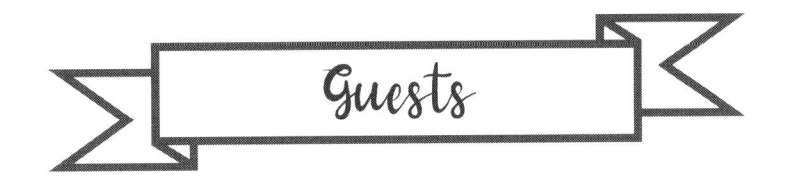

Advice for parents

_____
_____
_____

Wishes for baby

_____
_____
_____

Guests

Name and relationship to parents

_____
_____

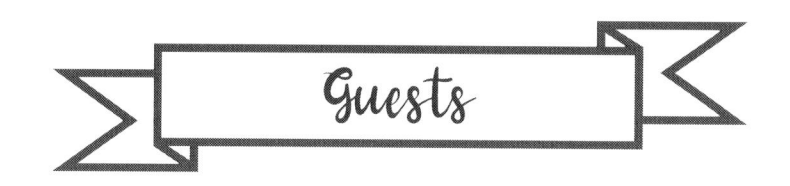

Advice for parents

_____
_____
_____
_____

Wishes for baby

_____
_____
_____
_____

Guests

Name and relationship to parents

_____

_____

Advice for parents

_____

_____

_____

Wishes for baby

_____

_____

_____

Guests

Name and relationship to parents

_____

_____

Advice for parents

_____

_____

_____

Wishes for baby

_____

_____

_____

Guests

Name and relationship to parents

_____
_____

Advice for parents

_____
_____
_____

Wishes for baby

_____
_____
_____

Guests

Name and relationship to parents

_____

_____

Advice for parents

_____

_____

_____

_____

Wishes for baby

_____

_____

_____

_____

Guests

Name and relationship to parents

_____
_____

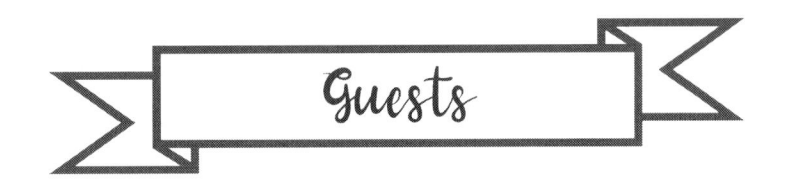

Advice for parents

_____
_____
_____
_____

Wishes for baby

_____
_____
_____
_____

Guests

Name and relationship to parents

_____
_____

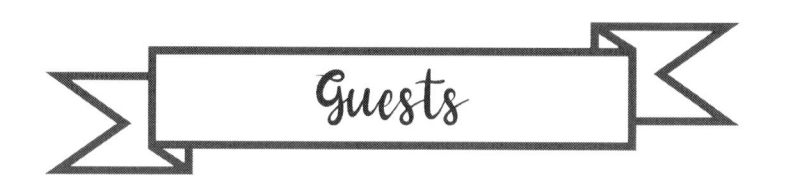

Advice for parents

_____
_____
_____

Wishes for baby

_____
_____
_____

Guests

Name and relationship to parents

_____
_____

Advice for parents

_____
_____
_____

Wishes for baby

_____
_____
_____

Guests

Name and relationship to parents

_____
_____

Advice for parents

_____
_____
_____

Wishes for baby

_____
_____
_____

Guests

Name and relationship to parents

_____

_____

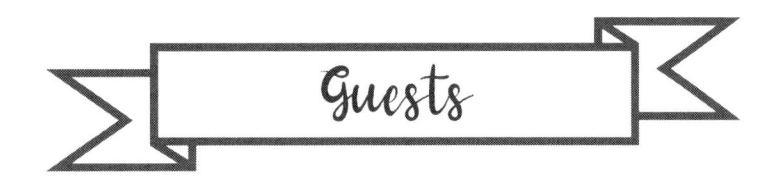

Advice for parents

_____

_____

_____

Wishes for baby

_____

_____

_____

Guests

Name and relationship to parents

_____
_____

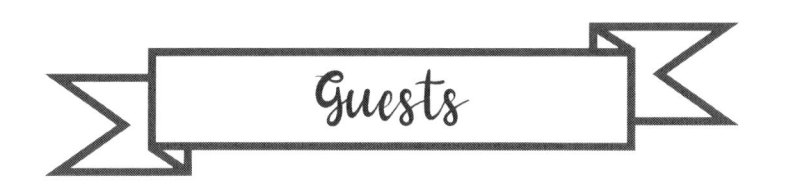

Advice for parents

_____
_____
_____

Wishes for baby

_____
_____
_____

Guests

Name and relationship to parents

_____
_____

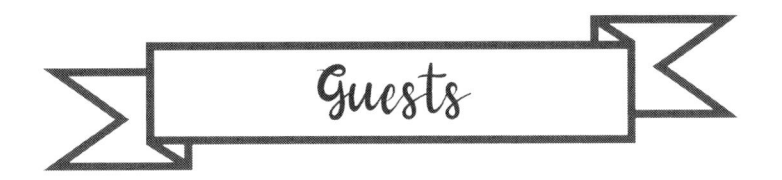

Advice for parents

_____
_____
_____

Wishes for baby

_____
_____
_____

Guests

Name and relationship to parents

_____

_____

Advice for parents

_____

_____

_____

Wishes for baby

_____

_____

_____

Guests

Name and relationship to parents

_____
_____

Advice for parents

_____
_____
_____

Wishes for baby

_____
_____
_____

Guests

Name and relationship to parents

_____

_____

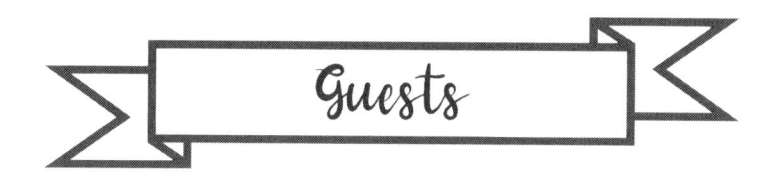

Advice for parents

_____

_____

_____

Wishes for baby

_____

_____

_____

Guests

Name and relationship to parents

_____

_____

Advice for parents

_____

_____

_____

Wishes for baby

_____

_____

_____

Guests

Name and relationship to parents

_____
_____

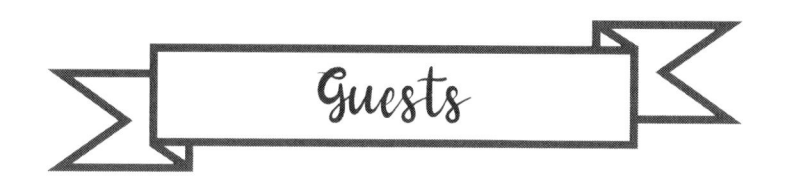

Advice for parents

_____
_____
_____

Wishes for baby

_____
_____
_____

Guests

Name and relationship to parents

_____

_____

Advice for parents

_____

_____

_____

Wishes for baby

_____

_____

_____

Guests

Name and relationship to parents

_____

_____

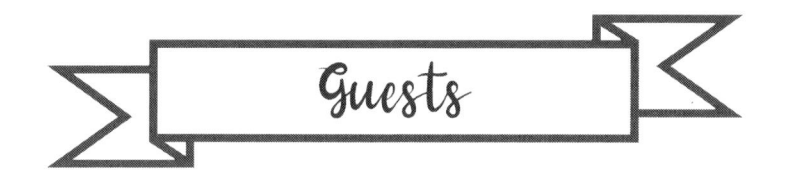

Advice for parents

_____

_____

_____

Wishes for baby

_____

_____

_____

Guests

Name and relationship to parents

_____

_____

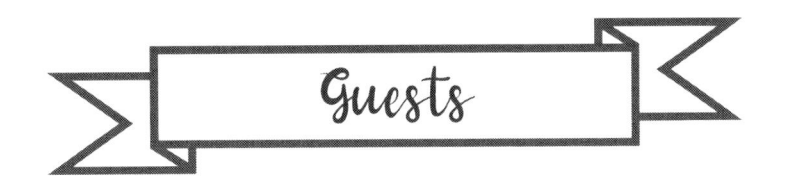

Advice for parents

_____

_____

_____

Wishes for baby

_____

_____

_____

Guests

Name and relationship to parents

_____
_____

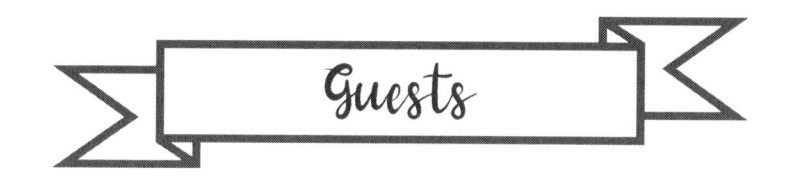

Advice for parents

_____
_____
_____

Wishes for baby

_____
_____
_____

Guests

Name and relationship to parents

_____

_____

Advice for parents

_____

_____

_____

Wishes for baby

_____

_____

_____

Guests

Name and relationship to parents

_____
_____

Advice for parents

_____
_____
_____
_____

Wishes for baby

_____
_____
_____
_____

Guests

Name and relationship to parents

_____

_____

Advice for parents

_____

_____

_____

Wishes for baby

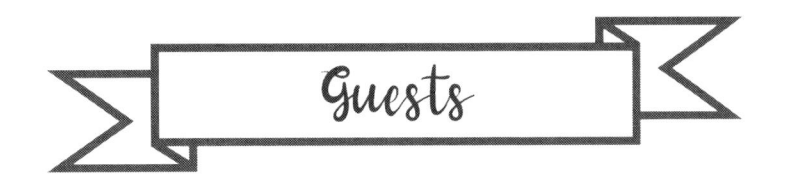

_____

_____

_____

Guests

Name and relationship to parents

_____
_____

Advice for parents

_____
_____
_____

Wishes for baby

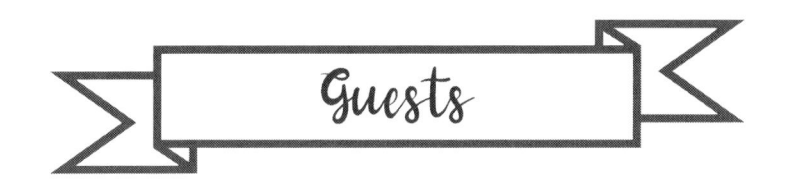

_____
_____
_____

Guests

Name and relationship to parents

_____
_____

Advice for parents

_____
_____
_____

Wishes for baby

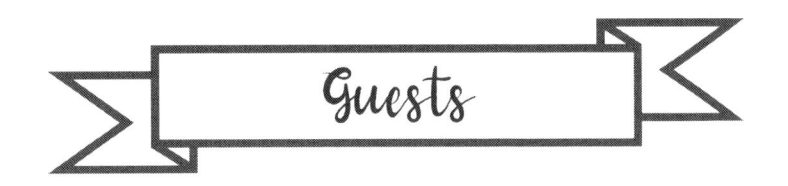

_____
_____
_____

Guests

Name and relationship to parents

_____

_____

Advice for parents

_____

_____

_____

Wishes for baby

_____

_____

_____

Gift log

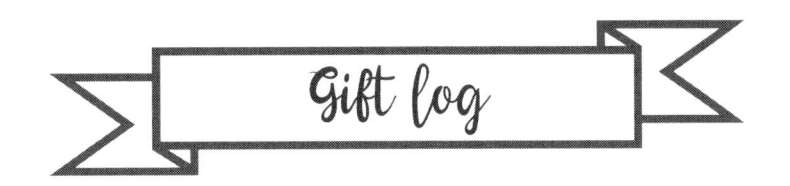

Gift	Given by

Gift log

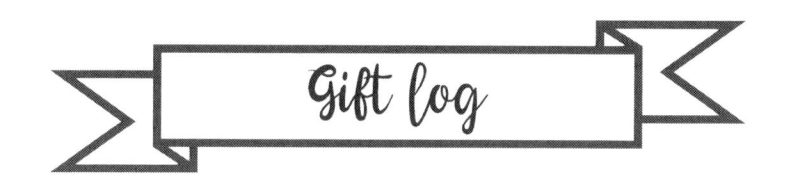

Gift	Given by

Gift log

Gift   Given by

Gift log

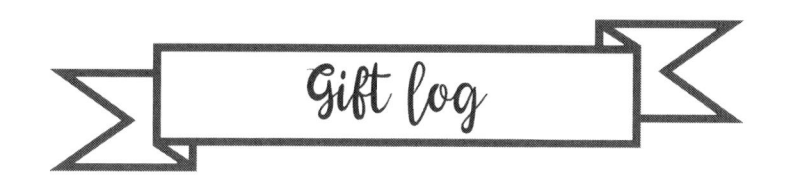

Gift	Given by

Gift log

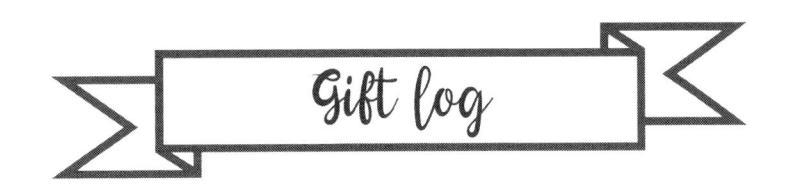

Gift	Given by

Gift log

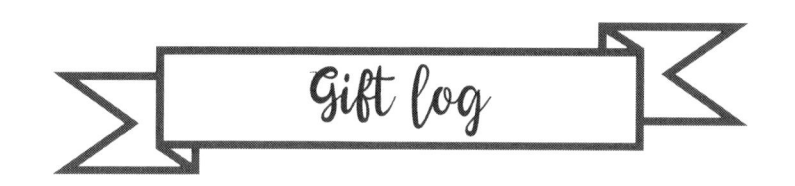

Gift	Given by

Gift log

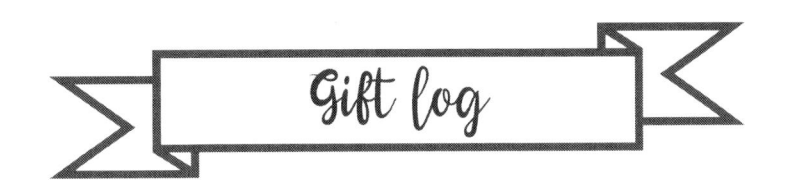

Gift	Given by

Gift log

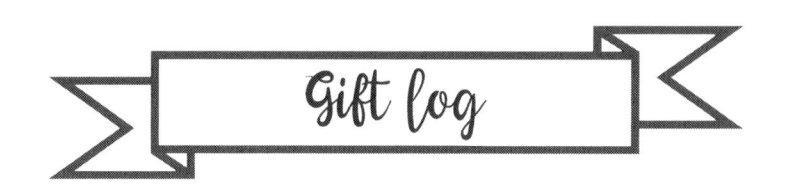

Gift	Given by

Gift log

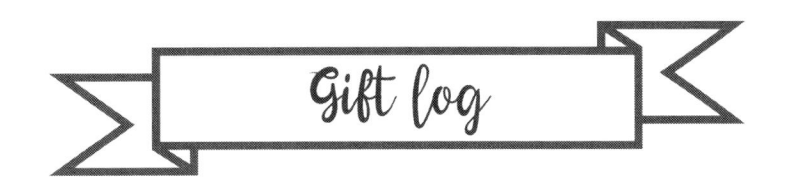

Gift	Given by
_____	_____
_____	_____
_____	_____
_____	_____
_____	_____
_____	_____
_____	_____
_____	_____
_____	_____
_____	_____
_____	_____
_____	_____

Gift log

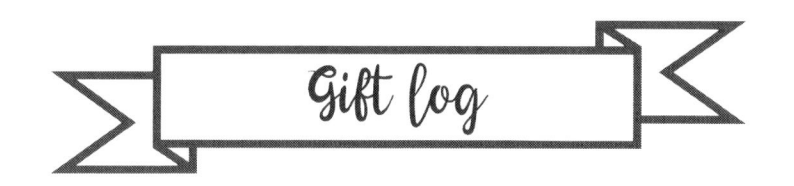

Gift	Given by

Special memories

Special memories

Special memories

Special memories

Special memories

Special memories

Special memories

Special memories

Special memories

Special memories

Made in the USA
Monee, IL
17 February 2025